RADIOFREQUENCY SKIN TIGHTENING FOR BEGINNERS

Comprehensive Guide To Non-Surgical Facial And Body Contouring, Wrinkle Reduction, And Advanced Techniques For Effective Results

DR SAWYER DIEGO

ABOUT THE BOOK

A thorough guide to comprehending and utilizing the advantages of radiofrequency (RF) technology in skin care is provided by Radiofrequency Skin Tightening for Beginners. For anyone seeking non-invasive ways to improve the firmness and appearance of their skin, this book is a vital resource.

After reading a thoughtful introduction to radiofrequency skin tightening, readers will understand the basic ideas underlying this ground-breaking procedure. It looks at how RF radiation can efficiently target the skin's deep layers, promoting the creation of collagen and providing long-term advantages.

This guide is valuable since it covers the fundamentals of radiofrequency skin tightening in great depth. The book provides a strong foundation for comprehending the transforming impacts of radiofrequency (RF) therapies, ranging from the historical development of RF treatments to the complex mechanics of RF radiation on skin tissues. Additionally, it sets RF apart from other popular skincare procedures by describing its special advantages and adaptability to a variety of skin types. The importance of safety cannot be overstated. It includes crucial rules for safe and efficient use, as well as things to think about while selecting RF devices and controlling treatment expectations.

There is helpful guidance on planning, carrying out, and recovering from care for individuals thinking about getting professional help or choosing to use at-home gadgets. This covers thorough instructions for utilizing RF equipment at home safely and successfully.

It also offers insights into professional treatment protocols and how to choose trained practitioners. The book also discusses how to combine radiofrequency (RF) with other skincare techniques, such as chemical peels, and dermal fillers, to provide a comprehensive strategy for getting the best results.

The guide addresses frequent worries and misunderstandings while guiding readers through possible side effects, risk-reduction techniques, and long-term maintenance procedures. It clarifies anticipated results and treatment duration, highlighting the significance of creating a customized skincare regimen following treatment. Readers' confidence in radiofrequency skin tightening procedures is fostered by real-life testimonials and professional insights, which enable them to make well-informed decisions regarding their skincare journey.

Throughout, FAQs address frequently asked questions concerning RF treatments, making sure readers have the information they need to make confident decisions regarding their skincare. Through an exploration of the science and real-world uses of radiofrequency skin tightening, this book encourages proactive learning and the pursuit of youthful, refreshed skin."

CHAPTER ONE

RADIOFREQUENCY SKIN TIGHTENING OVERVIEW

WHAT IS SKIN TIGHTENING THROUGH RADIOFREQUENCY (RF)?

A non-invasive cosmetic procedure called radiofrequency (RF) skin tightening aims to rejuvenate the skin by increasing the production of collagen, a protein that gives the skin structure but whose production declines with age, resulting in wrinkles and sagging. RF treatments work by heating the deeper layers of the skin with radiofrequency energy, which causes collagen fibers to contract and gradually encourages the production of new collagen, giving the skin a firmer, smoother texture and a reduction in fine lines and wrinkles.

A handheld device is used to apply controlled radiofrequency energy to the skin during an RF treatment session. The energy heats the targeted area without harming the skin's outer layer, or epidermis.

Because there is little chance of burns or changes in pigmentation, RF treatments are safe for all skin types and colors. Usually, several sessions are needed to get the best results; each session lasts between thirty and sixty minutes, depending on the area being treated.

With little to no downtime following treatment, patients can resume their daily activities right away. RF skin tightening is commonly used on areas such as the face, neck, abdomen, and thighs to improve skin laxity and enhance overall skin tone and texture. The procedure is generally well-tolerated, with patients reporting a warming sensation as the RF energy penetrates the skin.

RF SKIN TIGHTENING BENEFITS

For those looking for non-surgical rejuvenation, radiofrequency (RF) skin tightening has many advantages. The first is that it can tighten and firm skin without invasive surgery or a lengthy recovery period. Unlike surgical procedures such as facelifts,

RF treatments are non-invasive and do not involve incisions, which lowers the risk of complications and recovery time.

RF energy targets deep layers of the skin where collagen resides, promoting long-term skin health and elasticity. This results in a natural-looking enhancement that continues to improve over several months after the initial treatment sessions. Another important benefit is the gradual improvement in skin tone and texture that occurs with ongoing collagen production.

Overall, the benefits of radiofrequency skin tightening include smoother, firmer skin with a more youthful appearance and enhanced self-confidence.

It can also be tailored to target specific areas of concern, such as loose skin on the abdomen or fine lines around the eyes. This versatility makes it a versatile option for addressing various signs of aging and skin laxity across different body areas.

HOW RADIOFREQUENCY IS APPLIED TO SKIN

To achieve a noticeable improvement in skin tightness and firmness after the first treatment session, radiofrequency energy is delivered deep into the skin's dermal layers, where collagen fibers are located. The RF energy heats these tissues, causing them to contract and tighten immediately.

With time, RF energy also activates fibroblasts, which are the cells that produce collagen. When collagen is produced more readily, skin rejuvenation occurs gradually, and improvements last for several months after treatment. Because RF skin tightening has the dual benefits of immediate tightening and long-term collagen remodeling, it is a popular option for people who want to look younger without undergoing surgery.

Most patients describe the procedure as warm and comfortable, with no need for anesthesia or numbing creams.

The procedure is carried out using a handheld device that emits RF energy in controlled pulses or continuous waves, depending on the specific treatment protocol. The device is systematically moved over the treatment area to ensure an even distribution of heat and consistent results.

SAFETY POINTS TO REMEMBER

Since there are no incisions or injections involved, there is less chance of infection or scarring, and the controlled delivery of RF energy ensures that only targeted tissues are affected, leaving the surrounding skin and organs unharmed, RF skin tightening is generally regarded as safe, with minimal risks and side effects when performed by a trained professional.

Like any cosmetic procedure, RF skin tightening can have some potential side effects, though these usually go away within a few hours to a few days. To maximize results and minimize potential side effects, it's important to adhere to your provider's post-treatment care instructions. Temporary redness, swelling, or mild discomforts are some of the effects that could occur after RF skin tightening.

A qualified healthcare provider or dermatologist should be consulted before undergoing RF skin tightening to ensure suitability and safety. Patients with certain medical conditions, such as autoimmune disorders or severe skin diseases, may not be suitable candidates for RF skin tightening. Pregnant women and people with pacemakers or metal implants near the treatment area should also avoid RF treatments due to safety concerns.

BY WHOM IS RF SKIN TIGHTENING BENEFICIAL?

RF skin tightening is appropriate for a broad spectrum of people who want to improve skin laxity and improve the overall appearance of their skin. It is especially helpful for people who are dealing with early signs of aging, like fine lines, wrinkles, and mild skin sagging.

RF treatments can be customized to target specific issues on different body parts, making them useful for both face and body rejuvenation.

Ideal candidates are generally in good overall health and have mild to moderate skin laxity that can benefit from collagen stimulation and tissue tightening effects of radiofrequency energy. Candidates should have realistic expectations about the results, understanding that multiple treatment sessions may be needed to achieve optimal improvement.

A qualified cosmetic dermatologist or aesthetic practitioner can help determine whether RF skin tightening is the right option based on individual skin concerns and goals. Those seeking a non-invasive alternative to surgical procedures like facelifts or body lifts may find RF skin tightening particularly appealing. The procedure offers gradual, natural-looking results with minimal downtime, allowing patients to resume their daily activities immediately after treatment.

CHAPTER TWO

PRINCIPLES OF SKIN TIGHTENING USING RADIOFREQUENCY

AN EXPLANATION OF RF SKIN TIGHTENING ORIGINS

To rejuvenate the skin, radiofrequency (RF) skin tightening tightens the underlying tissues of the skin and stimulates the production of collagen. This non-invasive cosmetic procedure has become popular because it effectively reduces fine lines, wrinkles, and sagging skin without the need for surgery. Originally, RF technology was used in physical therapy to heat deep tissue, but as technology advanced, it was adapted for use in aesthetic medicine.

Today's RF skin tightening procedures function by applying radiofrequency (RF) energy to the dermis and subcutaneous layers, which are the deeper layers of the skin. This energy heats the dermis, which is rich in collagen, causing an instant contraction and subsequently stimulating the production of collagen over time. The end effect is smoother, firmer skin with improved elasticity and a decrease in visible signs of aging. Since RF treatments are generally comfortable and require no downtime, they are a popular option for people looking for non-surgical skin rejuvenation.

THE SKIN'S MECHANISM OF RF ENERGY

The mechanism of radiofrequency (RF) energy involves applying controlled heat to the deeper layers of the skin. RF devices use electromagnetic waves that pass through the skin and transform into thermal energy. This heat stimulates the fibroblasts, which are cells that produce collagen. The skin tightens and becomes more resilient as new collagen forms and collagen fibers contract. RF energy is safer than lasers because it penetrates deeper into the skin without harming the epidermis.

In an RF treatment session, the RF device is moved over the treatment area in a systematic pattern; patients usually experience a warming sensation as the device delivers energy to the skin; most people tolerate the procedure well; no anesthesia is needed; results are gradual and continue to improve over several weeks as collagen remodeling occurs; depending on the individual's skin condition and treatment goals, multiple sessions may be recommended for optimal results.

VARIOUS RF DEVICE TYPES

Different types of radiofrequency (RF) devices are used in cosmetic procedures; these include bipolar, multipolar, and monopolar RF systems. Bipolar RF devices target superficial layers of the skin by using two electrodes to deliver energy between them; multipolar RF devices use multiple electrodes to deliver energy uniformly and controllably, enhancing collagen production and skin tightening across a range of depths.

The selection of a device and treatment parameters is customized to the patient's concerns and skin condition, ensuring safe and effective results.

For example, monopolar RF may be preferred for body contouring and cellulite reduction, while bipolar or multipolar RF is frequently used for facial skin tightening and wrinkle reduction. Each type of RF device offers unique advantages based on the treatment area and desired outcomes.

WHAT SETS RF APART FROM OTHER SKIN TREATMENTS

When it comes to its mechanism of action and target areas, radiofrequency (RF) skin tightening is different from other skin treatments like laser therapy and chemical peels. Lasers use light energy to target specific pigments or skin imperfections, whereas RF energy heats the deeper layers of the skin to stimulate collagen production and tighten tissues. Because of this, RF treatments are appropriate for people with darker skin tones who may be at risk of pigment changes with laser treatments.

These characteristics make radiofrequency (RF) skin tightening a flexible option for people seeking to achieve smoother, firmer skin without invasive procedures. Unlike chemical peels, which exfoliate the skin's surface to improve texture and tone, RF treatments concentrate on remodeling collagen and improving skin elasticity from within.

RF is non-ablative, meaning it does not remove or damage the outer layer of skin, allowing for quicker recovery and minimal downtime.

COMPREHENDING COLLAGEN PRODUCTION AND SKIN LAYERS

Understanding the structure of the skin and how collagen production contributes to the youthful appearance of the skin is essential to understanding the effectiveness of radiofrequency skin tightening. The skin is composed of three main layers: the dermis, the epidermis, and subcutaneous tissue. Collagen, a protein abundant in the dermis, gives the skin structural support and elasticity. Collagen production decreases with age and environmental factors, resulting in skin laxity and wrinkle formation.

Understanding these skin dynamics helps patients appreciate how RF treatments can effectively rejuvenate their skin's appearance without invasive measures. RF energy specifically targets the dermis and subcutaneous layers, where collagen fibers reside. By heating these layers, RF treatments induce collagen contraction and stimulate fibroblasts to produce new collagen, improving skin firmness and elasticity over time and restoring a more youthful appearance.

For those who are new to RF skin tightening, all of these topics—definition and history, RF energy mechanism, device types, distinctions from other treatments, and comprehension of skin layers—offer a thorough introduction. With this knowledge, people are better equipped to choose their skincare products and aesthetic procedures, resulting in the best possible results for skin that is healthier and looks younger.

CHAPTER THREE

SELECTING THE PROPER RF DEVICE

THINGS TO TAKE INTO ACCOUNT WHILE CHOOSING AN RF DEVICE

Several important considerations should be made when choosing an RF (Radiofrequency) device for skin tightening. Firstly, the technology itself should be the primary consideration; seek out devices that make use of cutting-edge RF technology, which is well-known for its efficacy in stimulating collagen production and tightening the skin. Secondly, take into account the frequency range and energy levels the device operates on, as these factors determine the depth of penetration into the skin layers, which in turn affects the treatment results.

The device's portability and size are important considerations, particularly if you plan to use it at home or in various treatment settings. Make sure the device is FDA-cleared or CE-marked for safety and efficacy, indicating that it has met strict regulatory standards. Beginners should choose devices with user-friendly interfaces, clear controls, and ergonomic designs that ensure comfortable handling during treatments.

Finally, take into account the brand's reputation and reviews of the device. To evaluate a product's dependability, durability, and overall performance, looks for professional and customer reviews. Reputable brands frequently offer better warranty options and customer support—two things that are critical for troubleshooting and long-term satisfaction.

COMMON RF PRODUCTS AVAILABLE

Several RF devices are well-known for their effectiveness and easy-to-use features. The Tripollar STOP X is a well-liked option because of its small size and TriPollar RF technology, which provides concentrated radiofrequency energy for skin tightening and rejuvenation.

It can be used for both facial and body treatments and shows noticeable effects after repeated use.

Another noteworthy device is the Venus Legacy, which is valued for its adaptability in treating different body areas and skin types, consistently producing minimal discomfort, and reducing cellulite by combining Multi-Polar RF and Pulsed Electro Magnetic Fields (PEMF).

With its ergonomic design and simple operation, the Silk'n Titan is a great choice for beginners looking to incorporate radiofrequency (RF) treatments into their skincare routines.

VALUE FOR MONEY AND BUDGETARY ISSUES

Budget is an important consideration when choosing an RF device. Prices can differ significantly based on technology, brand reputation, and included features. Higher-end devices may cost more but frequently have more advanced settings and treatment possibilities.

Budget considerations should be balanced with the device's value and long-term benefits for beginners. While some mid-range options offer a good balance between affordability and performance, making them suitable for home use without compromising on results, cheaper devices might not offer the same level of effectiveness or durability as their more expensive counterparts.

When evaluating the whole worth, account for extra expenses like maintenance, warranty coverage, and replacement parts (such as treatment tips). Some businesses improve the entire value proposition by offering financing alternatives or package deals that include skincare goods or accessories.

FEATURES OF SAFETY TO CONSIDER

When choosing an RF device for skin tightening, safety should always come first. Look for devices that have integrated safety features like temperature sensors, automated shut-off mechanisms, and energy-setting adjustments.

These features help prevent overheating and guarantee a comfortable treatment while minimizing the risk of burns or skin damage.

Devices with intuitive interfaces and clear safety indicators make it easier for beginners to operate them correctly and safely. Choose devices that have been clinically tested and approved for their safety and efficacy by regulatory bodies like the FDA or CE. Read user manuals thoroughly to understand proper usage guidelines and safety precautions.

Always conduct a patch test before beginning treatment to evaluate the skin's reaction to the RF energy and determine the patient's tolerance. Speaking with a skincare expert or dermatologist can also offer helpful advice on device safety and customized treatment regimens. Take into consideration devices that have contact cooling systems or cooling gels that improve comfort during treatments, especially for sensitive skin areas.

COMPREHENDING THE SPECIFICATIONS AND CONFIGURATIONS OF DEVICES

Achieving the best possible treatment results requires an understanding of the specifications and settings of an RF device. Pay particular attention to parameters like treatment modes (continuous or pulsed), energy output levels (measured in Joules or Watts), and frequency range (measured in MHz). These settings determine the depth of penetration and intensity of RF energy delivered to the skin.

If your device offers customizable options for more targeted treatments, familiarize yourself with how to adjust settings manually. For beginners, devices with pre-set treatment programs or guided modes simplify the process by automatically adjusting settings based on the area being treated and skin type. This lowers the risk of errors and ensures consistent results with each session.

The specifications of your device also include information about how long treatments should last, how often sessions should be spaced apart, and what outcomes can be expected. Pay close attention to the instructions provided by the manufacturer to get the most out of your treatments and reduce the possibility of negative side effects. Monitoring your skin's changes over time will help you make necessary adjustments to the settings or consult a professional for continuous improvements.

Beginners can utilize RF devices with confidence to get tighter, smoother skin with customized treatments based on their personal skincare goals by being aware of these specs and settings.

CHAPTER FOUR

GETTING READY FOR AN RF PROCEDURE

MEETING WITH A SKIN SPECIALIST OR DERMATOLOGIST

A consultation with a dermatologist or skin specialist is essential before beginning any RF treatment. This first step guarantees that the procedure is appropriate for your skin type and addresses any specific concerns you may have. The dermatologist will examine your skin, go over your medical history, determine whether you are a good candidate for RF skin tightening, and go over the possible risks and benefits of the treatment.

To determine the best course of action, the dermatologist will usually examine the areas that are of concern, such as fine lines, wrinkles, or sagging skin. They may suggest radiofrequency skin tightening as a non-invasive option to improve skin firmness and texture.

Additionally, you will be able to ask questions about the procedure, including its effectiveness, expected results, and any instructions for post-treatment care. By speaking with a professional, you will receive individualized insights into how radiofrequency treatment can improve the health and appearance of your skin, ensuring a customized strategy for reaching your aesthetic objectives.

Having a consultation also helps you build a relationship with your dermatologist or skin specialist and develop confidence in the course of treatment. This proactive measure helps you get ready both physically and mentally for the procedure and guarantees that you will receive comprehensive care for the duration of your RF skin-tightening journey.

SKINCARE ROUTINE BEFORE TREATMENT

To ensure that the RF energy can penetrate the skin evenly during the treatment session, your dermatologist will likely recommend a structured skincare regimen that you should follow to maximize the effectiveness of the procedure and minimize any potential side effects. Generally, you will be advised to thoroughly cleanse your skin using a gentle cleanser to remove any impurities, makeup, or sunscreen.

Apart from cleansing, your dermatologist might advise you to use hydrating skincare products with antioxidants or hyaluronic acid, which nourish and moisturize the skin, improving its general health and resilience. You should also wear sunscreen every day to protect your skin from UV rays, which can interfere with the results of RF treatments.

In addition, following a pre-treatment skincare routine helps prepare the skin for the procedure and speeds up the healing process.

With regular practice, you may maximize the results of radiofrequency skin tightening and get smoother, firmer skin with better tone and texture.

WHAT TO ANTICIPATE FROM THE PROCESS

In a dermatologist's office or skincare clinic, you will be made to feel comfortable in a treatment chair or bed during the RF skin tightening procedure. The treatment usually starts with the application of a conductive gel to the treatment area, which helps to facilitate RF energy delivery and ensures uniform heating of the skin. Next, a handheld device that emits controlled radiofrequency energy into the deeper layers of the skin will be used by the dermatologist or trained technician.

As the RF energy targets and stimulates the regeneration of collagen fibers in the skin, you might feel warm or slightly heated. The procedure is generally well-tolerated, with most patients reporting minimal discomfort.

The length of the session varies depending on the size of the treatment area and your individual skincare goals, but it usually lasts between 30 and 60 minutes.

There is usually no downtime associated with radiofrequency skin tightening, so you can resume your daily activities right away. Over the next few weeks, you might notice gradual improvements in skin texture and firmness as collagen remodeling keeps your skin supple. Throughout the procedure, the dermatologist or technician will monitor your skin's response to ensure optimal energy delivery and treatment efficacy.

CONTROLLING EXPECTATIONS AND ASSIGNING REASONABLE OBJECTIVES

While RF technology can effectively improve skin firmness and reduce wrinkles, it is important to recognize that results may vary depending on individual skin characteristics and treatment adherence.

Setting realistic goals entails talking with your dermatologist about your desired outcomes and matching them with realistic expectations based on your skin's condition and response to treatment.

Managing expectations before undergoing RF skin tightening involves understanding the treatment's capabilities and limitations.

The anticipated timeframe for noticeable improvements is usually several weeks to months after treatment; to maximize outcomes, keep lines of communication open and adhere to any post-procedure instructions given by your healthcare provider. Moreover, embracing a healthy skincare regimen and lifestyle choices, like drinking plenty of water and shielding your skin from the sun, can further enhance the long-term advantages of radiofrequency skin tightening.

You can extend the longevity of your results and look younger and more refreshed by keeping reasonable expectations and following recommended skincare practices. Schedule follow-up appointments with your dermatologist so that treatment plans can be adjusted and progress can be evaluated, so you can continue to be satisfied with the results of your radiofrequency skin tightening.

WARNING SIGNS AND EXCLUSIONS

It's important to know about any precautions and contraindications before having RF skin tightening. People with certain medical conditions, like active infections, autoimmune disorders, or skin conditions like dermatitis or eczema, might not be good candidates for RF treatment. Women who are pregnant or nursing should also wait to have RF procedures done until after giving birth or lactation.

In addition, patients with a history of keloid scars or excessive skin laxity might need more specialized treatment plans or other options depending on their individual needs. Your dermatologist will perform a thorough evaluation at the initial consultation to determine any contraindications and guarantee your safety during treatment.

You must inform your healthcare provider of any pertinent medical history, current medications, and skincare product allergies to reduce risks and maximize treatment results.

You can undergo RF skin tightening with confidence if you prioritize safety precautions and follow professional guidance. Your dermatologist will prioritize your skin health and overall well-being. Additionally, adhering to post-procedure instructions, such as avoiding direct sun exposure and applying recommended skincare products, is crucial for supporting skin healing and minimizing potential side effects.

CHAPTER FIVE

HOW TO DO AT-HOME RF SKIN TIGHTENING

HOW-TO MANUAL FOR USING RF DEVICES AT HOME

Applying conductive gel to the treatment area to improve radiofrequency wave penetration is one of the most important safety precautions when using home RF devices for skin tightening. After that, follow the manufacturer's instructions to adjust the device's settings, usually starting with lower intensity levels to see how your skin responds.

After treating each area for the recommended amount of time, wipe off any remaining gel gently and hydrate the skin with a calming moisturizer or serum. Regular use, usually recommended 2-3 times per week, helps maintain results over time.

After treatment, move the RF device slowly and evenly over the skin in circular motions, ensuring consistent contact and coverage.

Most devices emit a gentle warmth or tingling sensation during use, which is normal.

SAFETY RECOMMENDATIONS FOR DOMESTIC USE

It is important to ensure safety when using home radiofrequency treatments. Before beginning, carefully read and follow the user manual. Avoid using RF devices near the eyes, open wounds, or irritated skin. Before beginning a full treatment, conduct a patch test on a small area of skin to check for any adverse reactions or sensitivity. Wipe the device clean with a damp cloth after each use. Store it in a cool, dry place out of children's reach.

Keep an eye on how your skin responds both during and after each session. If you notice any unusual reactions, redness, or extreme discomfort, stop using the device and see a dermatologist. Gradually increase the intensity settings as you get more comfortable with it and your skin's tolerance. Consistency and patience are essential to seeing noticeable improvements in the texture and tightness of your skin.

UPKEEP AND SANITIZATION OF DOMESTIC APPLIANCES

Your home radio frequency (RF) device will work better and last longer if you take care of it. To clean and maintain it, wipe the treatment head with a damp cloth after each use. Don't use harsh chemicals or alcohol-based cleaners as these could cause damage to the device's components. Store the device in its original case or a designated storage area to keep dust and moisture out.

You can continue to enjoy safe and effective skin tightening treatments at home by maintaining your RF device by these guidelines. Frequently check the device for any signs of wear or malfunction. If you notice unusual noises, overheating, or erratic performance, contact the manufacturer for guidance. Periodically inspect the power cord and plug to ensure they are intact and free of damage.

THE FREQUENCY AND LENGTH OF AT-HOME THERAPIES

The number and length of home radiofrequency treatments should be determined by your skin's response and treatment objectives. Begin with two to three sessions a week, adjusting the frequency and duration according to your skin's tolerance and the recommended usage guidelines of the device. Each session lasts for fifteen to thirty minutes and targets specific areas of concern, such as the face, neck, or abdomen.

Consistency is key to achieving long-term benefits from home RF treatments, so establish a routine that fits your schedule and skincare goals.

Gradually increase or decrease treatment intervals based on improvements in skin tightness and texture. Track your skin's response to each session to determine the best frequency for maintaining results

.

TRACKING OUTCOMES AND MODIFYING TREATMENT INTENSITY

Take before and after pictures to track progress and compare results from session to session. Pay attention to how your skin feels and looks immediately after treatment and in the days that follow. Track changes in skin firmness, texture, and overall appearance over time.

During sessions, adjust the intensity of the treatment based on your skin's response and comfort level. To achieve the best-tightening effects, start with lower intensity settings and gradually increase as tolerated. If you notice a plateauing or minimal improvement in the results, see a skincare professional for personalized advice or other treatment options. To ensure continued progress and satisfaction with your home RF device, regularly reevaluate your skincare routine and treatment plan.

CHAPTER SIX

EXPERT RADIOFREQUENCY TREATMENT METHODS

AN OVERVIEW OF EXPERT RADIOFREQUENCY TREATMENTS

Professional radiofrequency (RF) treatments are non-invasive procedures that use radiofrequency energy to improve skin elasticity and reduce wrinkles. By stimulating collagen production and tightening existing collagen fibers in the skin's deeper layers, controlled RF energy is delivered into the skin's layers, helping to achieve smoother, firmer skin without the need for surgery. RF treatments are typically used on areas such as the face, neck, and body to address signs of aging and skin laxity.

Treatment times vary depending on the area being treated but generally range from 20 to 60 minutes per session. The procedure starts with the application of a conductive gel on the treatment area to enhance RF energy penetration and protect the skin's surface.

Then, the RF device is moved over the skin in a predetermined pattern, delivering thermal energy to the underlying tissues. Patients may feel a warming sensation or mild discomfort during the procedure, which is usually well-tolerated without anesthesia.

Results are gradual, with noticeable improvements in skin tightness and texture becoming apparent over several weeks as collagen remodeling takes effect; multiple sessions spaced several weeks apart are often recommended to achieve optimal results; overall, RF treatments offer a safe and effective option for people seeking non-surgical skin rejuvenation with minimal downtime. Following the procedure, patients may experience mild redness or swelling, which usually resolves within a few hours to a few days.

LOCATING A CLINIC OR QUALIFIED PRACTITIONER

Look for qualified professionals who have received specific training in RF technology and are board-certified. This will ensure that the practitioner follows industry standards and best practices. When considering professional RF treatments, it is important to find a qualified practitioner or clinic with expertise in cosmetic dermatology or aesthetic medicine. Start by researching local providers who specialize in RF procedures and have a track record of delivering safe and effective results.

A consultation is a good idea before booking a treatment because it allows you to talk to the practitioner about your expectations, goals, and any concerns you may have. The practitioner will evaluate your skin condition, go over treatment options, and work with you to create a customized plan.

You should also ask about the practitioner's experience with RF treatments, including how many procedures they perform each year and if they have any before and after pictures of past patients.

A positive experience and satisfactory results from your RF treatment sessions can be ensured by checking that the clinic maintains proper accreditation and adheres to strict hygiene protocols. You should also find out what kind of RF device they use, as modern technology can improve treatment outcomes and safety.

EXPENSES AND COVERAGE BY INSURANCE

Professional radiofrequency (RF) treatments can be expensive depending on several factors, including the location of the clinic, the size of the treatment area, and the number of sessions needed. Generally speaking, a single RF session can cost anywhere from several hundred to several thousand dollars.

It is important to ask about pricing during your consultation and go over any financing options or package deals that might be available to reduce the cost of treatments.

Though some clinics may offer financing plans or payment options to help manage upfront costs, it's important to note that cosmetic procedures like radiofrequency (RF) treatments are typically not covered by health insurance plans because they are considered elective. Make sure to clarify payment terms and cancellation policies before committing to treatment to avoid any unexpected expenses.

While cost is a factor, safety, and effectiveness should come first when deciding where to receive radiofrequency treatments for the best results and peace of mind.

When comparing prices between different clinics, take into account the overall value based on the practitioner's experience, the caliber of the facility, and the outcomes attained by prior patients.

AFTERCARE AND RECUPERATION

Following post-treatment care instructions is crucial to maximizing results and minimizing potential side effects following professional radiofrequency (RF) treatments. Following the procedure, the treated area may appear slightly red or swollen, resembling a mild sunburn. This is normal and usually goes away in a few hours to a few days.

Apply any post-procedure skincare products—such as light cleansers and moisturizers—as directed by your practitioner to aid in the healing process. Keep the treated area out of the sun and wear high-SPF sunscreen to prevent UV damage. Don't use harsh skincare products or get other cosmetic procedures done until your skin has completely healed.

Follow-up appointments as scheduled to monitor your progress and discuss any concerns with your practitioner.

By following post-treatment guidelines, you can extend the longevity of your results and experience smoother, firmer skin in the long run. Maintain a healthy skincare routine and stay hydrated to support collagen production and skin recovery.

When evaluating the efficacy of professional radiofrequency treatments, one must consider the gradual changes in skin texture, firmness, and overall appearance that usually occur in the weeks following each treatment session. Your physician will monitor your progress during follow-up appointments and may suggest additional sessions to reach the desired result.

Compare before-and-after photos to objectively evaluate changes in your skin's condition during follow-up evaluations. Talk to your practitioner about any areas that you would like to see further improvement in, or that you would like to see addressed.

Your practitioner may modify your treatment plan or suggest complementary procedures to enhance results, like combining RF treatments with other skincare modalities.

To sustain and extend the benefits of radiofrequency (RF) therapy, you should plan for follow-up treatments at intervals that your practitioner recommends. Maintaining skin tightness and promoting collagen production over time require regularity in treatment sessions; by taking an active role in your skin care regimen and adhering to your practitioner's recommendations, you can be satisfied with the outcomes of professional RF treatments for a long time.

CHAPTER SEVEN

RF IN ADDITION TO OTHER SKIN TREATMENTS

COMBINED THERAPIES FOR BETTER OUTCOMES

To maximize the benefits of radiofrequency (RF) skin tightening treatments for that seeking enhanced skin rejuvenation, it is important to investigate complementary options that can amplify results. One such complementary option is the integration of RF with micro-needling, a technique that stimulates collagen production and improves skin texture. Patients who combine RF with micro-needling can achieve deeper penetration of RF energy into the skin layers, maximizing the benefits of collagen remodeling and tightening effects.

This combined approach is especially useful for minimizing fine lines, wrinkles, and acne scars, ultimately leading to smoother, more youthful-looking skin.

Moreover, combining RF with lymphatic drainage techniques or facial massages can further improve circulation, decrease fluid retention, and accelerate the removal of toxins from the treated areas, resulting in a more radiant complexion and longer-lasting results. LED light therapy is another useful combination with RF treatments, as it speeds up healing after the procedure and enhances cellular metabolism. LED therapy can be applied right after RF to calm the skin, reduce redness, and promote collagen synthesis.

Combining radiofrequency (RF) treatments with chemical peels can result in significant improvements for patients with uneven skin tone or pigmentation. Chemical peels exfoliate the skin's outer layers, improving the absorption of RF energy and improving the consistency of skin tone and texture. This combined approach effectively treats both pigmentation concerns and textural irregularities, leaving patients with skin that is clearer, smoother, and more radiant.

RADIATION THERAPY AND DERMAL FILLERS

Combining dermal fillers with radiofrequency (RF) skin tightening procedures provides a complete solution for those who want both skin tightening and volume restoration at the same time.

Dermal fillers, which are usually made of hyaluronic acid or other collagen-stimulating substances, are injected into specific areas to contour facial features and restore lost volume. RF treatments tighten loose skin and stimulate the production of collagen, so they work in concert to improve facial rejuvenation.

RF energy helps to tighten the skin around the injected filler, reducing the appearance of wrinkles and fine lines while promoting long-term collagen regeneration. This dual approach not only provides immediate volume enhancement but also improves skin texture and elasticity over time, offering patients a natural and youthful appearance.

Dermal fillers and RF treatments work particularly well together to address nasolabial folds, marionette lines, and hollow areas under the eyes.

A customized treatment plan that maximizes the synergy between dermal fillers and RF technology for improved facial contouring and skin tightening can be obtained by patients by consulting with a qualified cosmetic practitioner.

This combined approach guarantees comprehensive results that are both natural-looking and long-lasting. Individual aesthetic goals and concerns can be targeted, and customized treatment plans can be created to address them.

BOTOX AND RADIATION THERAPY

The dual-action approach to facial rejuvenation that results from combining Botox injections with radiofrequency (RF) skin tightening treatments targets both dynamic wrinkles and skin laxity. Botox is a neurotoxin that temporarily relaxes the facial muscles that cause expression lines; it is strategically injected to smooth out wrinkles like frown lines, forehead lines, and crow's feet. When combined with RF treatments, which tighten loose skin and stimulate collagen production, the result is a comprehensive solution for achieving smoother, firmer skin texture.

Combining Botox and RF technology works especially well for areas of the face that are prone to dynamic wrinkles and loss of elasticity.

The deep penetration of RF energy into the dermal layers improves skin tightness and enhances collagen synthesis, while Botox targets and relaxes underlying facial muscles. This two-pronged approach reduces wrinkles while also preventing new ones from forming, giving the appearance of renewed youth.

Additionally, combining Botox with RF treatments enables customized treatment regimens that target particular aesthetic issues and facial regions. Whether augmenting the outcomes of RF skin tightening with

Botox injections or the other way around, patients can attain results that are natural-looking and improve facial contours and overall skin texture. Through consultation with a qualified cosmetic specialist, patients can receive a customized strategy that optimizes the synergistic effects of Botox and RF technology for the best possible facial rejuvenation.

CHEMICAL EXTRACTION AND RADIOFREQUENCY

Chemical peels, which use acids like glycolic acid or salicylic acid to exfoliate the skin and improve texture, tone, and clarity, are one method of skin rejuvenation that targets both surface imperfections and underlying skin laxity.

When combined with RF treatments, which tighten loose skin and stimulate collagen production, the result is an improved overall appearance and firmness of the skin.

Chemical peels help RF energy enter the dermal layers of the skin more deeply and effectively by removing dead cells and encouraging cell turnover. This synergy improves overall skin tone, minimizes fine lines, wrinkles, and acne scars, and promotes collagen remodeling. Those who want complete skin rejuvenation with little downtime can benefit most from the combination of chemical peels and RF treatments.

Incorporating chemical peels with radiofrequency (RF) technology further enables customized treatment plans that are suited to specific skin concerns and goals.

Whether treating pigmentation problems, acne scars, or signs of aging, this combined approach guarantees comprehensive improvements in skin texture, tone, and elasticity. Patients can receive a customized regimen that optimizes the synergistic effects of chemical peels and RF treatments for optimal skin rejuvenation by speaking with a qualified skincare professional.

TAILORING THERAPY PROGRAMS TO INDIVIDUAL REQUIREMENTS

To effectively address individual aesthetic goals and skin conditions, treatment plans that combine RF skin tightening with complementary therapies must be customized.

Since each patient has a unique skin type, set of concerns, and desired outcome, a personalized approach to treatment is required. Healthcare providers can create a customized plan by taking into account variables like skin elasticity, texture, and particular areas of concern.

Assessing the degree of skin laxity and choosing the right frequency and intensity of radiofrequency treatments are important components of creating personalized treatment regimens.

People with mild to moderate skin laxity might benefit from a course of RF treatments plus dermal fillers or microneedling to gradually tighten and volumize their skin.

People with more prominent wrinkles or deeper signs of aging might benefit from a course of RF treatments plus chemical peels or Botox injections to target both dynamic wrinkles and skin texture.

Additionally, post-treatment care and maintenance are customized to ensure patient satisfaction and long-lasting results. Combining skincare regimens to support sun protection, hydration, and collagen production improves the results of combined radiofrequency treatments.

Follow-up appointments allow for modifications to the treatment plan based on individual response and changing aesthetic goals, ensuring ongoing improvement in the quality and appearance of the skin.

Through close collaboration with skilled medical professionals, patients can create customized treatment regimens that combine radiofrequency skin tightening with other therapies in a way that optimizes outcomes and suits their requirements.

This individualized approach not only addresses individual aesthetic concerns but also encourages general skin health and rejuvenation, enabling patients to confidently and successfully achieve their desired outcomes.

CHAPTER EIGHT

HANDLING RISKS AND SIDE EFFECTS

COMMON RF SKIN TIGHTENING SIDE EFFECTS

Beginners should be aware of the common side effects of radiofrequency (RF) skin tightening, which is generally safe but can include temporary redness and mild swelling at the treatment site, which usually goes away in a few hours, some clients experience a warm sensation during the procedure, which is normal as the RF energy penetrates the skin layers, and rarely, but usually not very often, slight bruising.

To minimize discomfort and lower the risk of adverse reactions, practitioners frequently apply cooling gels or use cooling devices before, during, and after the RF treatment.

Novices must advise their clients about these possible side effects in advance so they are prepared for what to expect after treatment.

Appropriate aftercare, such as avoiding sun exposure and using gentle skin care products, can also help in effectively managing these common side effects.

Understanding these typical side effects and how to manage them is essential for ensuring that clients have a positive experience with radiofrequency skin tightening procedures. Practitioners can guarantee a more seamless and fulfilling treatment outcome by educating clients and using appropriate techniques.

RISKS IN THE SHORT- AND LONG-TERM

Even though radiofrequency skin tightening is generally thought to be safe, there are some significant short- and long-term risks to be aware of. Shortly after the procedure, some patients may experience mild soreness or sensitivity in the treated area. In rare instances, more serious side effects like burns, blisters, or pigmentation changes can happen, particularly if the patient has previously had skin conditions or the procedure is not done correctly.

To minimize long-term risks, beginners should make sure they have a thorough understanding of the equipment and techniques used in RF skin tightening. Appropriate energy levels and monitoring client responses during treatment can significantly reduce the likelihood of adverse effects. Long-term risks include potential scarring or infection if post-treatment care instructions are not followed diligently.

Before undergoing RF skin tightening, practitioners should thoroughly evaluate each client's medical history and skin condition to reduce these risks. It is crucial to minimize negative outcomes and advance safety in practice by educating clients about potential risks and making sure they understand the significance of adhering to aftercare instructions.

REDUCING RISKS WITH APPROPRIATE METHODS

Practitioners must follow correct techniques and safety procedures to mitigate the risks associated with radiofrequency skin tightening. The device must be calibrated appropriately for each client's skin type and treatment area to prevent burns or discomfort. New users should receive comprehensive instruction on how to operate radiofrequency devices safely and effectively, including knowledge of the best energy settings and treatment durations for various skin conditions.

Proper placement of the RF device and steady hand movements also help to reduce the risk of uneven heating or skin damage. Using appropriate cooling methods during treatment also helps to control the skin's temperature and minimize discomfort. Practitioners should continuously monitor the client's response to the treatment and adjust settings accordingly to ensure consistent and safe delivery of RF energy.

Beginners can improve patient satisfaction and reduce unfavorable reactions during radiofrequency skin tightening procedures by emphasizing safety and using best practices in technique.

Ongoing professional development and staying current with industry standards also help practitioners provide high-quality treatments with lower risks.

WHEN TO GET MEDICAL HELP

Practitioners and clients need to know when to seek medical attention following radiofrequency skin tightening. Although minor side effects such as redness and swelling are common and usually go away on their own, persistent or severe symptoms like intense pain, excessive swelling, or signs of infection should be immediately followed by a visit with a doctor. Patients who have had keloid scarring in the past or who have sensitive skin should be especially watchful and report any unexpected reactions as soon as possible.

To avoid complications and guarantee that any adverse reactions that may arise after the procedure are appropriately treated, practitioners should instruct their clients on the warning signs that indicate a need for medical attention and give them clear instructions on how to get in touch with their office or seek emergency care if necessary.

Practitioners can help ensure a safe and positive experience for their clients by keeping lines of communication open and stressing the need to monitor the skin's response following radiofrequency skin tightening. Prompt intervention in the event of unusual symptoms adds to client safety and upholds the practitioner's expertise and commitment to client care.

TAKING CARE OF THE CLIENT FEARS AND ANXIETY

Enhancing the overall client experience requires addressing client concerns and anxiety before, during, and after radiofrequency skin tightening treatments. A lot of clients have concerns about the procedure's safety, possible side effects, or discomfort during treatment; practitioners can help by thoroughly explaining the procedure, including how radiofrequency energy works to tighten skin and stimulate collagen production.

Providing reassurance about the safety measures in place, such as using FDA-approved devices and adhering to strict hygiene protocols, can further reassure clients about the procedure's safety and efficacy. Fostering an environment of open communication allows clients to express their concerns and ask questions, which helps build trust and confidence in the practitioner.

To help clients feel more at ease during the treatment itself, practitioners can employ calming techniques like relaxing music or exercises. They can also improve the overall experience of treatment by explaining each step of the procedure as it happens and following up with the client to find out how comfortable they are.

Clients should receive clear instructions on what to do after a procedure, including what to expect in the days that follow and the significance of skincare routines. By offering contact information for any queries or concerns that may arise, the practitioner demonstrates their commitment to patient care and guarantees continued support.

Practitioners can provide a positive experience that increases client satisfaction and encourages long-term commitment by proactively addressing client problems and creating a supportive environment.

CHAPTER NINE

RESULTS AND LONG-TERM MAINTENANCE

CREATING A SKINCARE ROUTINE AFTER TREATMENT

Creating a post-treatment skincare routine that works is essential to preserving and improving results from radiofrequency (RF) skin tightening treatments. After your RF session, you should protect and hydrate your skin by using moisturizers and gentle cleansers that are appropriate for your skin type to prevent irritation. You can also use aloe vera or soothing gel to relieve any temporary redness or swelling.

Sunscreen with a high SPF is a must-have to protect your skin from UV damage, which can undermine the effects of radiation therapy and prematurely age the skin. In the days after treatment, combining products high in antioxidants can support skin healing and collagen production stimulated by radiofrequency (RF).

Consistency is key in skincare routines post-RF treatment, ensuring you nurture your skin daily with products that support its newly found firmness and elasticity. To maintain skin moisture levels and enhance the plumping effects of RF, think about incorporating hydrating masks or serums containing hyaluronic acid into your long-term skincare routine.

REGULARITY OF MAINTENANCE PROCEDURES

To sustain the advantages of radiofrequency skin tightening, it's important to know how often maintenance treatments should be scheduled. Although individual skin conditions and treatment regimens can affect outcomes, most practitioners suggest scheduling maintenance appointments every 4 to 6 months to allow for ongoing collagen remodeling and to preserve the skin's firmness and texture.

Regular maintenance helps counteract the natural aging process by consistently stimulating the production of collagen and elastin, and each maintenance treatment involves adjusting the RF energy to maintain or further improve results based on your skin's response and any changes in your aging process. These sessions are usually shorter than initial treatments but are essential to maintaining long-term benefits.

Monitoring the time between maintenance treatments is crucial for increasing the effectiveness of radiofrequency skin tightening. Speaking with a skincare expert guarantees customized scheduling that is in line with your skin's requirements and objectives, maximizing the durability of your results over time.

MONITORING AND RECORDING OUTCOMES OVER TIME

To evaluate the results and make adjustments to future treatment plans, you must monitor and record the evolution of your skin's response to radiofrequency (RF) treatments over time. To start, take clear, well-lit pictures of your skin from different perspectives before beginning RF therapy, making note of any areas that are of concern, such as wrinkles, sagging, or uneven texture.

Note any improvements or areas that may require additional attention during follow-up appointments. Observe changes in the firmness, elasticity, and general texture of your skin after each RF session. Keeping a skincare journal or digital record can help you track subtle changes and keep realistic expectations regarding your treatment outcomes.

As collagen continues to remodel and tighten the skin, you should be able to see noticeable improvements over time by comparing your original photos with current images. By keeping track of these changes, you will be better equipped to make decisions about future treatments and changes to your skincare routine that will ensure that you continue to be satisfied with the way your skin looks.

LIFESTYLE ELEMENTS THAT IMPACT RF OUTCOMES

Several lifestyle choices can impact the efficacy and durability of radiofrequency skin tightening outcomes. Eating a well-balanced diet high in antioxidants, vitamins, and vital nutrients promotes general skin health and amplifies the benefits of radiofrequency treatments. Staying adequately hydrated is also critical because it increases skin elasticity and helps with the healing process after radiofrequency sessions.

Smoking and excessive alcohol consumption can also compromise skin elasticity and collagen production, potentially decreasing the efficacy of RF treatments over time. Avoiding excessive sun exposure and using sunscreen daily is paramount to protecting your skin from UV damage, which can diminish the effects of RF and accelerate skin aging.

Prioritizing these lifestyle factors can help you maximize the longevity of your RF skin tightening results and maintain a youthful, rejuvenated appearance. Reducing inflammation and promoting cellular repair processes are two ways that managing stress through relaxation techniques or mindfulness practices can positively impact skin health. Regular exercise improves circulation, which contributes to healthy skin and enhances the results of RF treatments.

TAKING CARE OF CONCERNS ABOUT AGING AND CONTINUING CARE

Beyond radiofrequency treatments, addressing aging concerns and preserving optimal skin health necessitates a multifaceted approach. As you age, your skin demands change, requiring ongoing care and modifications to your skincare routine. By encouraging collagen synthesis and cellular turnover, anti-aging ingredients like retinoids or peptides can enhance the effects of RF.

Frequent consultations with a skincare specialist enable customized evaluations and suggestions based on your evolving skin concerns; they can offer guidance on cutting-edge skincare procedures or technologies that support radiofrequency (RF), like micro needling or laser therapies, to target particular signs of aging, like deep wrinkles or hyperpigmentation.

Consistent support for the health and appearance of your skin can be obtained by sticking to a sun protection regimen and implementing a thorough skincare routine that includes cleansing, moisturizing, and targeted treatments. You can effectively manage aging concerns and achieve long-lasting improvements in skin firmness, texture, and radiance by combining proactive skincare practices with periodic RF treatments.

CHAPTER TEN

FAQ ON RADIATION SKIN TIGHTENING

WHAT AGE IS BEST TO BEGIN RF TREATMENTS?

While there is no set age for RF (Radiofrequency) treatments, most people consider them in their late 20s to early 30s when collagen production naturally starts to decline and early signs of aging become noticeable.

The ideal age for beginning RF (Radiofrequency) treatments varies depending on individual skin concerns and goals. Generally, RF treatments are popular among adults who are beginning to experience signs of aging such as fine lines, wrinkles, and skin laxity.

The effectiveness of radiofrequency (RF) treatments can vary depending on skin condition and individual response, so it's important to consult with a skincare expert to determine the best-starting age based on individual skin concerns and goals. Older adults may seek RF to address existing wrinkles and skin sagging. Generally, RF treatments are safe for adults of various ages as long as they have realistic expectations and consult with a qualified dermatologist or skincare professional.

IS IT POSSIBLE TO COMBINE RF TREATMENTS WITH OTHER SKINCARE PRODUCTS?

RF treatments primarily target deeper layers of the skin to stimulate collagen production and improve skin tightness and texture; when combined with topical skincare products like moisturizers, serums, and sunscreens, they can optimize results and maintain skin health. Yes, RF treatments can enhance and complement other skincare products when used as part of a comprehensive skincare regimen.

Hyaluronic acid, peptides, and antioxidants are examples of ingredients found in skin care products that can support skin hydration, repair, and protection—all of which are critical for overall skin health. A skincare professional can recommend specific products that address individual skin concerns and complement RF treatments, thereby enhancing the overall results of the treatment regimen, before combining RF treatments with other skincare products to ensure compatibility and effectiveness.

ARE RADIOFREQUENCY TREATMENTS UNCOMFORTABLE?

The majority of people find radiofrequency (RF) treatments to be well-tolerated and not painful. Patients may feel their skin heated slightly during the procedure, but this is controlled and comfortable. Most modern RF devices have cooling mechanisms built in to help patients feel comfortable and minimize discomfort during treatment sessions.

A mild redness or sensitivity may rarely occur immediately following treatment, but these side effects usually go away quickly.

The sensation experienced during RF treatments can vary depending on the intensity settings used and individual pain thresholds. Some patients may describe a tingling or prickling sensation similar to a gentle massage.

WHAT'S THE DURATION OF RF RESULTS?

While results may be noticeable shortly after treatment, optimal outcomes typically develop gradually over several weeks to months as collagen remodeling continues. Generally, radiofrequency (RF) treatments stimulate collagen production and improve skin tightness, which can result in gradual and progressive improvements over time. The longevity of RF results can vary depending on individual skin characteristics, treatment parameters, and lifestyle factors.

The duration of RF results can be influenced by factors like sun exposure, skincare regimen, and overall skin health. Regular use of sunscreen and adherence to a recommended skincare routine can help extend the longevity of RF results and promote overall skin health. Follow-up treatments may be recommended periodically to sustain collagen production and address ongoing skin aging concerns.

ARE ALL SKIN TYPES SUITED FOR RF TREATMENT?

Unlike some laser treatments that may be limited by skin color, RF technology targets the deeper layers of the skin without affecting the outer layer, making it suitable for people with a variety of skin types and tones. Generally speaking, RF treatments are safe and effective for a wide range of skin types, including fair to dark skin tones.

To ensure that RF treatments are customized for optimal safety and effectiveness, individuals with varying skin types must consult with a qualified dermatologist or skincare professional. They can assess skin characteristics and determine the most appropriate treatment plan, taking into account factors such as skin type, sensitivity, and specific concerns. By choosing the appropriate RF devices and treatment parameters, skincare professionals can ensure that individuals with different skin types achieve the desired results while minimizing potential risks or side effects.

CHAPTER ELEVEN

FREQUENT FEARS AND ILLUSIONS

TAKING CARE OF RF DEVICE SAFETY ISSUES

Safety is the most important factor when it comes to radiofrequency (RF) skin tightening. A lot of newcomers may wonder if RF devices are safe to use at home or if there are any risks involved. You should know that, when used properly, RF devices for skin tightening are generally safe. They emit radiofrequency energy, which penetrates the skin to heat the underlying tissues, stimulating collagen production and tightening the skin. However, some safety precautions need to be followed, like using FDA-approved devices and making sure they are operated according to the manufacturer's instructions. Additionally, beginners should be aware of any potential side effects, which are usually minor and transient and can include temporary redness or mild discomfort.

Beginners should follow a skincare routine that includes moisturizing and sun protection to maintain skin health during and after RF treatments. By proactively addressing safety concerns and seeking professional advice, beginners can enjoy the benefits of RF skin tightening with peace of mind. A dermatologist or licensed skincare professional can assess your skin type and recommend the appropriate RF device. They can also guide how to use the device safely and effectively at home.

DISPELLING UNTRUTHS REGARDING RF SKIN TIGHTENING

There are a few common misconceptions about radiofrequency (RF) skin tightening that can be confusing to newcomers. Firstly, most people only feel a slight warmth during treatment; discomfort is usually mild and well-tolerated. Secondly, there is a misconception that RF skin tightening is only useful for severe cases of skin sagging. While RF is useful for tightening loose skin, it can also improve skin texture and firmness in milder cases of aging or laxity.

Debunking these myths will help beginners approach RF skin tightening with realistic expectations and confidence in its effectiveness and convenience. Another myth to dispel is the idea that RF treatments are expensive and only available in clinics. Thanks to technological advancements, there are now affordable and effective RF devices for home use, making skin tightening more accessible to a wider audience. Additionally, RF treatments are non-invasive, meaning there is no downtime or recovery period required, unlike surgical procedures.

RECOGNIZING THE VARIATIONS BETWEEN SURGICAL AND RADIOFREQUENCY PROCEDURES

RF skin tightening is not the same as surgical procedures like facelifts or neck lifts; for one thing, RF treatments are non-invasive and non-surgical, and they work by heating collagen fibers and stimulating the production of new collagen by delivering energy into the deeper layers of the skin; over time, this process gradually tightens and lifts the skin, with the results becoming more noticeable with repeated sessions.

While RF can provide noticeable improvements in skin laxity and texture, it may not produce the same dramatic results as surgery for severe sagging. As such, individuals considering RF should have realistic expectations and understand that multiple sessions may be needed to achieve optimal results.

Unlike surgery, RF treatments typically do not require downtime, allowing individuals to resume their daily activities immediately after treatment.

Beginners can decide whether RF skin tightening is right for them depending on their tastes and cosmetic goals by being aware of these differences. Personalized advice based on specific skin conditions and desired results can also be obtained by consulting with a competent skin care practitioner.

CUSTOMER TESTIMONIALS & FIRSTHAND ACCOUNTS

For those new to RF skin tightening, reading client testimonials and real-world accounts can be a great way to gain insight. A lot of people post about their experiences online, talking about various RF devices, treatment plans, and outcomes. These testimonies frequently emphasize how well RF works to improve skin firmness, minimize wrinkles, and improve overall texture.

Anecdotal evidence can also highlight the variation in outcomes between patients; although some may experience noticeable improvements following a few sessions, others may need additional treatments to reach their goals.

Testimonials also frequently highlight how simple it is to incorporate radiofrequency treatments into everyday routines due to the procedure's non-invasive nature and little to no downtime.

In the end, hearing from others who have had RF treatments can encourage confidence and well-informed decision-making. To that end, beginners should look for testimonials from reliable sources and forums where users discuss their experiences transparently. These accounts can provide realistic expectations and help beginners gauge whether RF skin tightening is aligned with their skincare goals.

ENCOURAGING SELF-ASSURANCE IN RF SKIN TIGHTENING METHODS

The science of radiofrequency (RF) skin tightening procedures and its benefits for skin rejuvenation must be understood to foster confidence in the procedure. RF stimulates collagen production and tightens loose tissues by delivering thermal energy deep into the skin.

Many people find this non-invasive approach appealing because it offers gradual but noticeable improvements without the risks associated with surgery.

Beginners can boost their confidence by educating themselves about the various types and functions of radiofrequency (RF) devices as well as the specific benefits they offer for different skin concerns. They can also reinforce their confidence in the safety and efficacy of RF by learning about clinical studies and research that support RF efficacy. Lastly, consulting a skincare or dermatologist can provide customized recommendations based on individual skin types and conditions.